GALLBLADDER DIET COOKBOOK

"51 Wholesome Recipes for a Happy Gallbladder: Nourish, Heal, and Thrive with Our Gallbladder-Friendly Cookbook and meal plan"

By

Linda A ivey

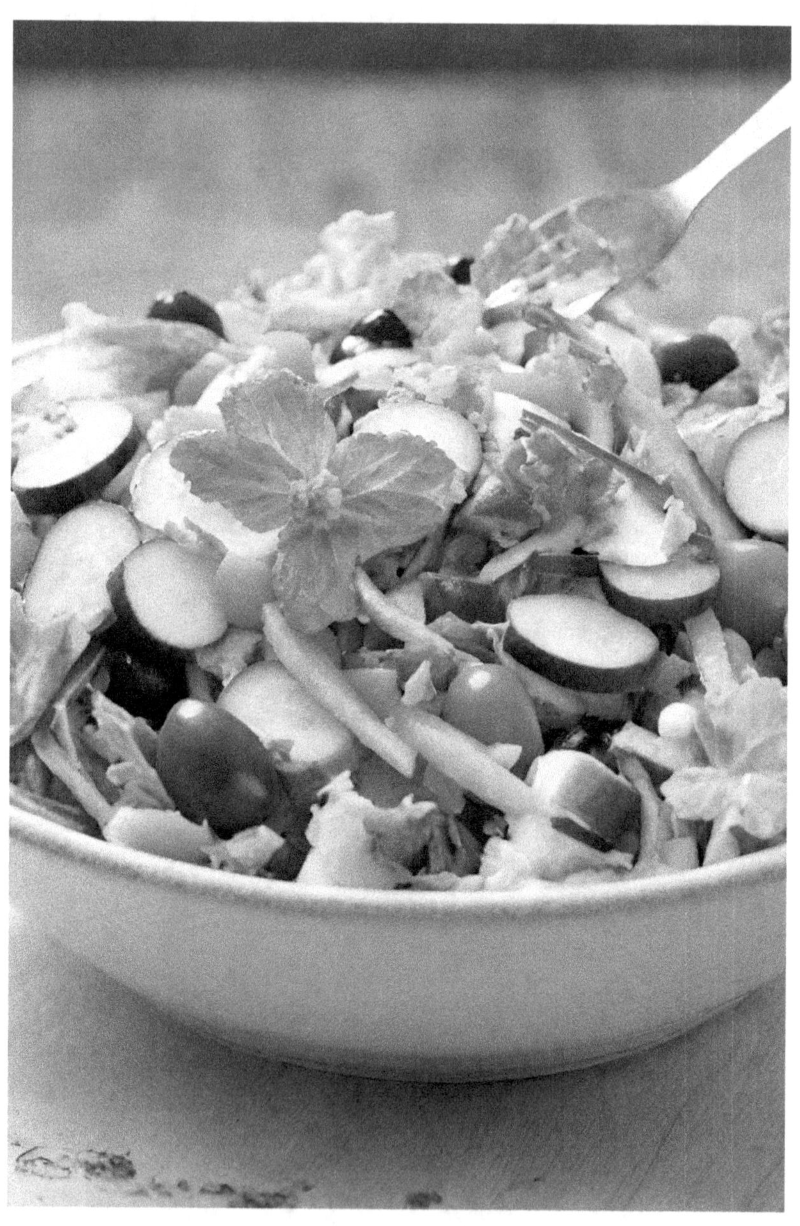

GAIN ACCESS TO MORE BOOKS FROM ME

Table of contents

Introduction

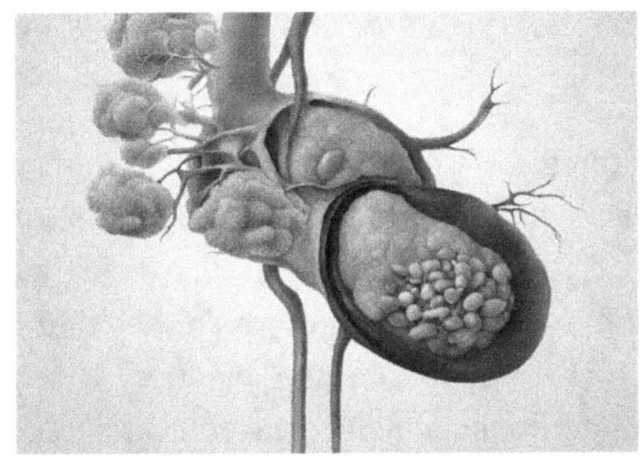

$\mathbf{W}$elcome to a culinary journey designed to transform the way you approach nourishment and well-being — "Wholesome Recipes for a Happy Gallbladder." This cookbook is more than just a collection of recipes; it's a guide to embracing a lifestyle that supports and cherishes your gallbladder health.

In these pages, we embark on a voyage to understand the intricate workings of the gallbladder, a resilient organ often overlooked until its harmony is disrupted. We'll delve into the significance of adopting a gallbladder-friendly diet and explore practical tips to seamlessly integrate this approach into your daily routine.

Imagine this introduction as the first step towards a healthier, more vibrant you. Picture a table filled with dishes that not only tantalize your taste buds but also nourish your body from within. The journey to gallbladder wellness begins here, and we invite you to savor every moment, every flavor, and every revelation along the way.

As we embark on this culinary expedition together, prepare to discover the art of crafting meals that not only respect the needs of your gallbladder but also celebrate the joy of wholesome eating. Whether you're seeking a fresh start or aiming to maintain the balance you've achieved, let this cookbook be your trusted companion on the path to a happy, gallbladder-friendly life.

Are you ready to embark on a flavorful adventure that transcends the boundaries of ordinary cookbooks? Turn the page, and let the transformation begin.

21 Tips for Adapting to the Gallbladder Diet

1. It is important to educate yourself on the activities of the gallbladder and how the choices you make about your food might affect its health.
2. ***Consult with a Healthcare Professional***: To customize dietary suggestions to your specific requirements, it is important to seek the expert guidance of a healthcare professional.

3. ***Hydrate with awareness***: Consuming an adequate amount of water improves digestion and aids in the prevention of gallstones.

4. ***Choose Healthy Fats***: Instead of consuming saturated and trans fats, choose healthy fats such as olive oil, avocados, and almonds while avoiding saturated fats.

5. ***Take Advantage of Lean Proteins***: Give lean proteins, such as fish, poultry, and alternatives derived from plants, the highest priority.

6. ***Include foods that are rich in fiber***, such as fruits, vegetables, and whole grains, in your diet to promote digestive health. Fiber is your friend.

7. To avoid overeating and to ensure that digestion is at its best, it is important to pay attention to the size of your portions.

8. Slow down, savor each meal, and pay attention to indicators associated with hunger and fullness while practicing mindful eating.

9. *Minimize Your Intake of Processed Foods*: Reduce your consumption of processed and refined foods, since they have been shown to contribute to inflammation.

10. *Experiment with Cooking Methods:* Explore baking, grilling, or steaming as healthier alternatives to frying.

11. *Be Wary of Spices:* Spices that are not too strong, such as ginger and turmeric, may be used to enhance flavor without straining the gallbladder.

12. *Consider Dietary Supplements*: Discuss with your healthcare practitioner if supplements like digestive enzymes may be useful.

13. ***Create Balanced Meals:*** Aim for a combination of proteins, healthy fats, and carbs in each meal.

14. ***Regular, Small Meals***: Opt for numerous, smaller meals throughout the day to aid the digestive process.

15. ***Mind Your Sugar Intake***: Choose natural sweeteners in moderation and minimize processed sugars.

16. ***caffeine Limit Caffeine and alcohol***: Both may influence gallbladder function, so reduce your usage.

17. ***Meal Planning:*** Prepare meals ahead of time to make healthier alternatives easily accessible.

18. ***Stay Active***: Regular exercise helps general health, including digestive function.

19. ***Manage Stress:*** Practice stress-reducing activities like meditation or yoga to support a healthy gut.

20. ***Listen to your body***: Pay attention to how your body reacts to various meals and change your diet appropriately.

21. ***Celebrate Progress:*** Acknowledge and celebrate the good adjustments you achieve on your gallbladder-friendly path.

Chapter 1

Gallbladder-Friendly Staples

In the area of a gallbladder-friendly diet, the choosing of fats is analogous to constructing a beautiful symphony — a harmonic balance of taste and health. Let's go on a sensory adventure as we study the art of picking fats that not only dance on your taste senses but also play a critical part in promoting gallbladder health.

1. Olive Oil Elegance: Picture the silky, golden shine of extra virgin olive oil, a master in the realm of good fats. Rich in monounsaturated fats, it not only lends a rich flavor to your foods but also supports gallbladder function.

2. Avocado, the Creamy Virtuoso: Imagine the velvety feel of ripe avocados, a virtuoso of healthy fats. Packed with monounsaturated fats and minerals, avocados give a creamy touch to your dishes while fostering gallbladder health.

3. Nutty Ensemble of Almonds and Walnuts: Envision the pleasant crunch of almonds and the earthy richness of walnuts — a nutty ensemble that contains important omega-3 fatty acids, delivering both taste and anti-inflammatory effects for the gallbladder.

4. Fatty Fish Ballet: Dive into the ocean of tastes with fatty fish like salmon and mackerel, the ballet dancers of omega-3 fatty acids. These fish not only delight your palette but also improve gallbladder health by lowering inflammation.

5. Coconut's Unique Melody: Transport yourself to a tropical paradise with the unique melody of coconut. Whether in the form of oil or milk, coconut adds a distinct taste character while supplying medium-chain triglycerides that are readily digested for gallbladder comfort.

6. Sesame Seed bliss: Picture the tiny sesame seeds scattered over your food, generating a fragrant bliss. Sesame seeds, rich in polyunsaturated fats, give a delicious crunch and help to gallbladder well-being.

Lean Proteins for Gallbladder Health

1. Poultry Poise: Imagine delicious, oven-roasted chicken or delicate turkey breast taking center stage. Poultry, with its lean profile, becomes the maestro, giving a protein-packed performance that promotes gallbladder health without losing flavor.

2. The Elegance of Fish Fillets: Picture a delicate fillet of salmon, trout, or cod, gleaming on your plate. Fatty salmon, high in omega-3 fatty acids, not only satisfies your taste senses but also orchestrates anti-inflammatory actions, encouraging harmony inside your gallbladder.

3. Plant-Based Symphonies: Envision a lively ensemble of lentils, chickpeas, and tofu delicately dancing in a vegetable stir-fry. Plant-based proteins help gallbladder health with their fiber content, supporting digestive comfort and presenting a diversity of delicious textures.

4. Lean Cuts of Red Meat: Picture a nicely grilled sirloin or tenderloin, displaying the skill of lean red meat cooking. While to be savored in moderation, these lean cuts contain high-quality protein, guaranteeing a full and gallbladder-friendly meal experience.

5. Eggcellent Performance: Dive into the variety of eggs, whether poached, scrambled, or in an omelet. Eggs give a protein-packed performance, rich in nutrients like choline that improve gallbladder function while giving a velvety texture to your culinary composition.

6. Dairy Delicacies: Envision the richness of Greek yogurt or cottage cheese joining the gourmet symphony. These dairy choices deliver lean protein, aiding gallbladder health while adding a wonderful creaminess to both sweet and savory recipes.

7. Quinoa Crescendo: Visualize a brilliant quinoa dish, decorated with colorful veggies. Quinoa, a plant-based complete protein, takes the stage, delivering a gluten-free and gallbladder-friendly option that adds both texture and nutritional depth to your dishes.

8. Seafood Serenade: Imagine the salty fragrance of shrimp or scallops sautéed to perfection. Seafood, dense in lean protein, brings a marine serenade that not only delights your taste sensations but also promotes gallbladder health via its nutrient-rich composition.

9. bird Tale of Tenderness: Picture a Thanksgiving feast with the star of the show — a succulent, oven-roasted bird. Turkey, especially the lean white flesh, conveys a narrative of softness, giving a protein-packed pleasure while adhering to gallbladder-friendly concepts.

10. Legume Lullaby: Envision a substantial stew cooking on the stove, containing an ensemble of beans. Legumes, especially kidney beans, black beans, and chickpeas, contribute to the diversity of protein alternatives, creating a tapestry of tastes and fiber that supports overall well-being.

11. Bison Ballad: Picture a lean bison burger on a whole-grain bun, a tribute to the lesser-known yet health-conscious meat possibilities. Bison, with its lean profile, provides a combination of taste and nutrition, promoting gallbladder health with its high-quality protein.

12. Edamame bonanza: Dive into a bowl of edamame, the young, colorful soybeans that give a protein-packed bonanza. Edamame, whether savored as a snack or integrated into recipes, provides both texture and gallbladder-friendly nutrients to the culinary stage.

13. Chicken Harmony in Stir-Fry: Imagine the sizzling of a stir-fry pan, showing strips of lean chicken amid a bright variety of veggies. Chicken, when harmoniously blended with a range of vegetables, becomes the melody of a gallbladder-friendly stir-fry, delivering both nutrition and taste.

In this symphony of lean proteins, let your culinary creativity go wild. Allow the savory tones of these protein sources to build a tapestry of enjoyment on your plate while helping the well-being of your gallbladder. As you explore these protein-rich alternatives, experience the range of tastes, textures, and nutrients that each item brings to the table, producing a culinary masterpiece that resonates with both taste and health.

High-Fiber Foods for Digestive Support

1. Kaleidoscope of veggies: Picture a variety of bright veggies—broccoli, bell peppers, carrots, and spinach—sautéed to perfection. This rainbow of vegetables delivers a spectrum of fiber that not only adds crunch and taste but also fosters a healthy digestive rhythm.

2. Quinoa Quilt: Imagine a quinoa salad garnished with cherry tomatoes, cucumbers, and fresh herbs. Quinoa, a versatile whole grain, offers a patchwork of fiber, giving it a pleasing texture that promotes digestive health while improving the nutritional profile of your dishes.

3. Berry Bliss Parfait: Imagine layers of Greek yogurt, granola, and a waterfall of mixed berries. Berries, with their natural sweetness and fiber content, form a pleasant parfait that not only fulfills your sweet desires but also supports a healthy digestive environment.

4. Legume Landscape: Visualize a hearty lentil soup simmering on the stove, highlighting the richness of legumes. Lentils, chickpeas, and black beans build a landscape of fiber, delivering both satiety and digestive support in a healthy and comforting dish.

5. Whole Grain Mosaic: Picture a platter covered with a mosaic of whole grains—brown rice, quinoa, and farro. Whole grains, with their fiber-rich composition, contribute to a mosaic that not only offers diversity to your meals but also supports a healthy digestive process.

6. Nutty Trail Mix: Dive into a dish loaded with almonds, walnuts, and pistachios. Nuts, with their crunchy texture and fiber content, make a trail mix that not only fulfills snack needs but also offers digestive assistance practically and pleasantly.

7. Avocado Avant-Garde: Envision avocado slices artfully arranged on whole-grain bread. Avocados, rich in both fiber and healthy fats, give an avant-garde accent to your meals, producing a creamy and satisfying experience that promotes digestive well-being.

8. Apple Orchard Symphony: Picture biting into a fresh apple or eating a warm dish of apple cinnamon porridge. Apples, with their soluble and insoluble fiber, lead an orchard symphony that not only delights your taste senses but also promotes digestive harmony.

Chapter 2

Delicious Breakfasts

- **Energizing Smoothie Bowls**

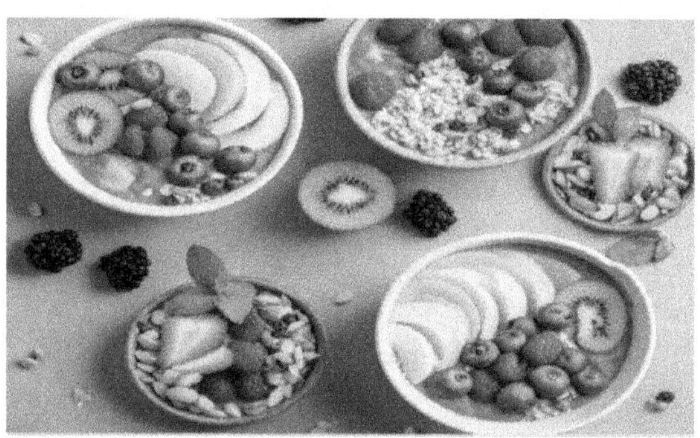

1. Berry Burst Bliss Bowl:

Ingredients:

- 1 cup mixed berries (strawberries, blueberries, raspberries)
- 1 frozen banana
- 1/2 cup Greek yogurt
- 1 tablespoon chia seeds
- 1/2 cup almond milk
- Toppings: Granola, sliced almonds, fresh berries

Instructions:

1. Blend the mixed berries, frozen banana, Greek yogurt, chia seeds, and almond milk until smooth.
2. Pour the smoothie into a bowl and top with granola, sliced almonds, and fresh berries for an extra burst of texture and flavor.

2. Tropical Paradise Power Bowl:

Ingredients:

- 1 cup pineapple chunks
- 1/2 cup mango chunks
- 1 frozen kiwi
- 1/2 cup coconut water
- 1 tablespoon hemp seeds
- Toppings: Toasted coconut, sliced kiwi, chia seeds

Instructions:

1. Blend pineapple, mango, frozen kiwi, coconut water, and hemp seeds until smooth.

2. Pour into a bowl and garnish with toasted coconut, sliced kiwi, and a sprinkle of chia seeds for a tropical energy boost.

3. Green Goddess Revitalizer Bowl:

Ingredients:

- 1 cup spinach leaves
- 1/2 cucumber, peeled and sliced
- 1/2 green apple, cored
- 1/2 avocado
- 1 tablespoon flaxseeds
- 1/2 cup coconut water
- Toppings: Sliced kiwi, pumpkin seeds, drizzle of honey

Instructions:

1. Blend spinach, cucumber, green apple, avocado, flaxseeds, and coconut water until velvety.
2. Pour into a bowl and top with sliced kiwi, pumpkin seeds, and a drizzle of honey for a green goddess-inspired bowl.

4. Chocolate Peanut Butter Protein Bowl:

Ingredients:

- 1 frozen banana
- 2 tablespoons peanut butter
- 1 scoop chocolate protein powder
- 1/2 cup almond milk
- 1 tablespoon cocoa powder
- Toppings: Sliced bananas, chopped peanuts, dark chocolate shavings

Instructions:

1. Blend frozen banana, peanut butter, chocolate protein powder, almond milk, and cocoa powder until creamy.
2. Transfer to a bowl and garnish with sliced bananas, chopped peanuts, and dark chocolate shavings for a protein-packed treat.

5. Mango Peach Sunrise Bowl:

Ingredients:

- 1 cup mango chunks
- 1/2 cup peach slices (fresh or frozen)
- 1/2 orange, peeled
- 1/2 cup coconut milk
- 1 tablespoon sunflower seeds

- Toppings: Fresh mango cubes, peach slices, a sprinkle of sunflower seeds

Instructions:

1. Blend mango, peach slices, orange, coconut milk, and sunflower seeds until smooth.
2. Pour into a bowl and top with fresh mango cubes, peach slices, and a sprinkle of sunflower seeds for a sunrise-inspired delight.

Revitalize your mornings and embrace the day with these energizing smoothie bowl recipes. Each spoonful is not just a burst of flavor but a nourishing symphony of vitamins, minerals, and energy-boosting goodness. Enjoy the journey to a revitalized and energized you!

- **Nutrient-Packed Oatmeal Varieties**

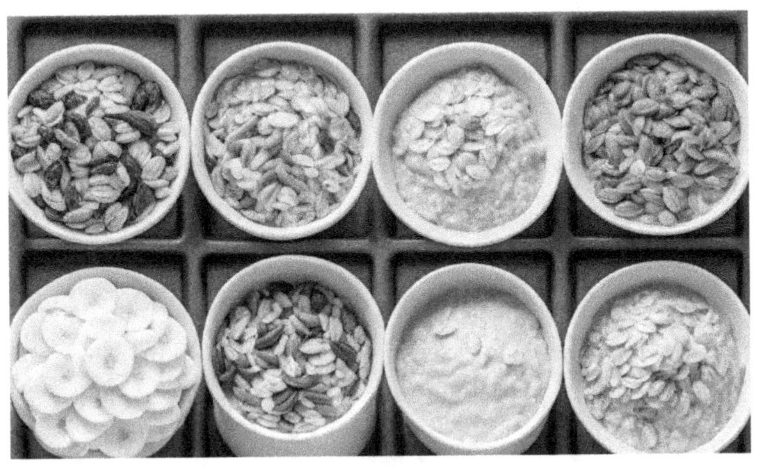

6. Classic Cinnamon Apple Oatmeal:

Ingredients:

- 1/2 cup old-fashioned oats
- 1 cup almond milk
- 1 apple, diced
- 1 teaspoon cinnamon
- Toppings: Sliced almonds, sprinkle of honey

Instructions:

1. In a saucepan, mix oats, almond milk, diced apple, and cinnamon.
2. Cook over medium heat, stirring periodically, forabout 5-7 minutes or until the oats are cooked and the mixture thickens.

3. Top with sliced almonds and a sprinkle of honey.

7. Triple Berry Bliss Oatmeal:

Ingredients:

- 1/2 cup rolled oats
- 1 cup water
- 1/2 cup mixed berries (strawberries, blueberries, raspberries)
- 1 tbsp chia seeds
- Toppings: Greek yogurt, more berries, a sprinkling of chia seeds

Instructions:

1. Combine oats, water, mixed berries, and chia seeds in a saucepan.
2. Cook over medium heat, stirring regularly, for 5-7 minutes or until the oats are cooked to your taste.
3. Top with a dollop of Greek yogurt, more berries, and a sprinkling of chia seeds.

8. Pumpkin Spice Power Oatmeal:

Ingredients:

- 1/2 cup steel-cut oats
- 1 cup milk of your choice
- 1/4 cup canned pumpkin puree
- 1/2 teaspoon pumpkin spice
- Toppings: Pepitas, a swirl of maple syrup

Instructions:

1. In a saucepan, add steel-cut oats, milk, pumpkin puree, and pumpkin spice.
2. Simmer over low heat, stirring periodically, for about 15-20 minutes or until the oats are soft and the mixture thickens.
3. Top with pepitas and a swirl of maple syrup.

9. Chocolate Banana Nut Oatmeal:

Ingredients:

- 1/2 cup quick-cooking oats
- 1 cup water
- 1 ripe banana, mashed
- 1 tablespoon cocoa powder
- Toppings: Sliced bananas, chopped walnuts, a drizzle of almond butter

Instructions:

1. Cook quick-cooking oats with water, mashed banana, and cocoa powder in a microwave-safe bowl for 2-3 minutes, stirring halfway through.
2. Top with sliced bananas, chopped walnuts, and a dab of almond butter.

10. Coconut Mango Chia Oatmeal:

Ingredients:

- 1/2 cup old-fashioned oats
- 1 cup coconut milk
- 1/2 cup cubed mango
- 1 tbsp chia seeds
- Toppings: Toasted coconut flakes, fresh mango cubes

Instructions:

1. Combine oats, coconut milk, chopped mango, and chia seeds in a saucepan.
2. Cook over medium heat, stirring periodically, for 5-7 minutes or until the oats are cooked and the mixture thickens.
3. Top with toasted coconut flakes and fresh mango cubes.

Adjust the cooking times depending on your liking for oatmeal consistency - whether you want it harder or creamier. Experiment with these nutrient-packed oatmeal variations to discover your ideal morning bowl of warmth and sustenance.

- **Light and Satisfying Breakfast Wraps**

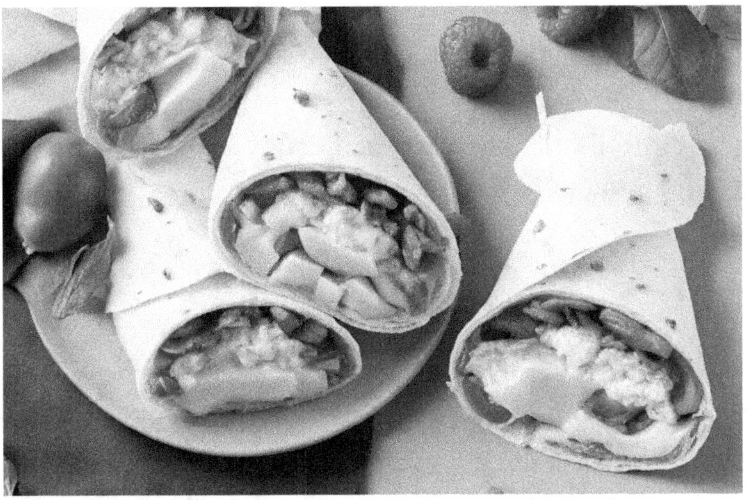

11.   Veggie-Packed Egg White Wrap:

Ingredients:

- 2 big egg whites
- 1 whole wheat tortilla
- 1/4 cup sliced bell peppers (any color)

- 1/4 cup chopped tomatoes
- Handful of spinach leaves
- Salt and pepper to taste

Instructions:

1. In a non-stick pan, cook egg whites over medium heat until set.
2. Place the cooked egg whites on a whole wheat tortilla.
3. Add chopped bell peppers, tomatoes, spinach leaves, and season with salt and pepper.
4. Roll up the wrap and enjoy a veggie-packed, protein-rich breakfast.

12. Greek Yogurt with Berry Delight:

Ingredients:

- 1 whole grain or spinach tortilla
- 1/2 cup Greek yogurt
- 1/2 cup mixed berries (strawberries, blueberries, raspberries)
- 1 tablespoon honey
- Granola for added crunch

Instructions:

1. Spread Greek yogurt evenly on the tortilla.
2. Add mixed berries and sprinkle with honey.
3. Sprinkle granola for some additional crunch.
4. Roll up the wrap and experience a mouthwatering blend of creamy yogurt and sweet berries.

13. Avocado and Turkey Breakfast Wrap:

Ingredients:

- 1 whole wheat or spinach tortilla
- 1/2 avocado, sliced 3 slices of turkey
- 1 egg, scrambled Salsa for a kick

Instructions:

1. Lay out the tortilla and lay sliced avocado in the middle.
2. Add turkey slices and scrambled egg on top.
3. Drizzle with salsa for extra taste.
4. Roll up the wrap for a protein-packed, avocado-infused morning delight.

14. Smoked Salmon with Cream Cheese Wrap:

Ingredients:

- 1 whole grain or multigrain tortilla
- 2 tablespoons cream cheese
- 2 ounces smoked salmon
- Red onion slices
- Capers for garnish

Instructions:

1. Spread cream cheese over the tortilla.
2. Layer smoked salmon and red onion slices.
3. Garnish with capers.
4. Roll up the wrap and bask in the wonderful blend of smoked salmon and creamy cheese.

15. Mango Tango Breakfast Wrap:

Ingredients:

- 1 coconut or plain tortilla
- 1/2 cup cottage cheese
- 1/2 ripe mango, chopped
- Handful of mint leaves, chopped
- Drizzle of honey

Instructions:

1. Spread cottage cheese evenly across the tortilla.
2. Add diced mango and chopped mint.
3. Drizzle with honey for sweetness.
4. Roll up the wrap and enjoy a tropical breakfast delight.

These light and tasty breakfast wraps not only give a lovely start to your day but also provide a healthy mix of nutrients to keep you nourished and content.

Chapter 3

Wholesome Lunches and Dinners

- **Flavorful Grilled Chicken and Fish Recipes**

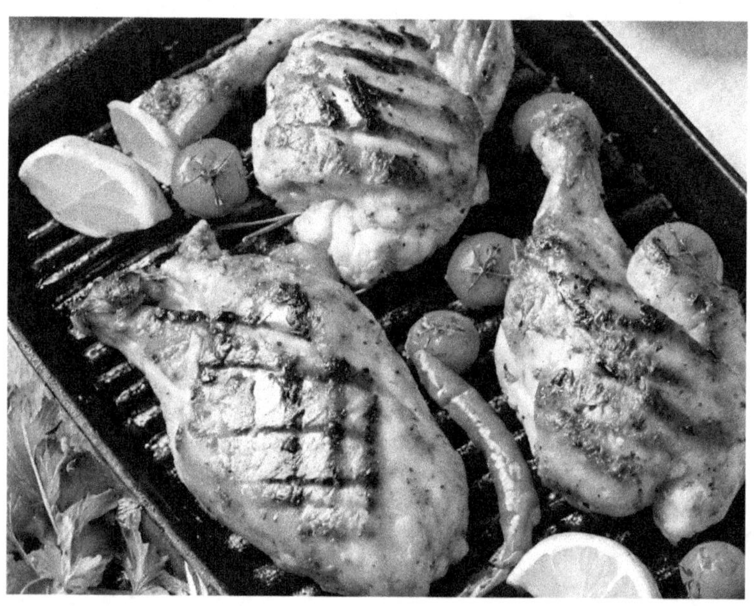

16. Grilled Lemon Herb Chicken:

Ingredients:

- 4 boneless, skinless chicken breasts
- 1/4 cup olive oil
- 2 teaspoons fresh lemon juice
- 2 cloves garlic, minced
- 1 teaspoon dried oregano
- 1 teaspoon dried thyme
- Salt and black pepper to taste

Instructions:

1. In a bowl, mix olive oil, lemon juice, minced garlic, oregano, thyme, salt, and pepper.
2. Marinate the chicken breasts in the marinade for at least 30 minutes.
3. Preheat the grill to medium-high heat.
4. Grill the chicken for 6–8 minutes per side, or until thoroughly done.
5. Serve with a squeeze of fresh lemon juice, and garnish with chopped herbs.

17. Honey Garlic Glazed Salmon:

Ingredients:

- 4 salmon fillets
- 1/4 cup soy sauce
- 2 tablespoons honey

- 1 tablespoon olive oil
- 2 cloves garlic, minced
- 1 teaspoon grated ginger
- Garnish with chopped green onions and sesame seeds.

Instructions:

1. In a small bowl, combine the soy sauce, honey, olive oil, chopped garlic, and grated ginger to prepare the marinade.
2. Marinate the salmon fillets for at least 20 minutes.
3. Preheat the grill to medium heat.
4. Grill the salmon for 4-5 minutes on each side, basting with the marinade.
5. Before serving, garnish with green onions diced and sesame seeds.

18. Cajun Spiced Grilled Chicken Thighs:

Ingredients:

- 8 bone-in, skin-on chicken thighs
- 2 tablespoons olive oil

- 2 teaspoons Cajun seasoning
- 1 teaspoon smoked paprika
- 1 teaspoon garlic powder
- 1 teaspoon onion powder
- Salt and cayenne pepper to taste

Instructions:

1. In a bowl, add olive oil, Cajun spice, smoked paprika, garlic powder, onion powder, salt, and cayenne pepper.
2. Rub the spice mixture over the chicken thighs, ensuring uniform covering.
3. Let the chicken marinate for at least 30 minutes.
4. Preheat the grill to medium-high heat.
5. Grill the chicken thighs for 15-20 minutes, rotating periodically, until thoroughly cooked and crispy.

19. Lemon Herb Grilled Tilapia:

Ingredients:

- 4 tilapia fillets
- 3 tablespoons olive oil
- 2 teaspoons fresh lemon juice
- 1 teaspoon dried thyme

- 1 teaspoon dried rosemary
- Salt and black pepper to taste

Instructions:

1. In a small bowl, mix olive oil, lemon juice, dried thyme, dried rosemary, salt, and black pepper.
2. Marinate the tilapia fillets for 15-20 minutes.
3. Preheat the grill to medium heat.
4. Grill the tilapia for 3-4 minutes on each side or until the fish flakes easily with a fork.
5. Serve with a squeeze of fresh lemon juice and extra herbs.

These tasty grilled chicken and fish dishes guarantee to make your meals a joyful experience. Whether you're a lover of spicy citrus, robust Cajun spices, or sweet honey glazes, these recipes provide a range of flavors to suit any pallet. Enjoy the grilling adventure and relish the tasty outcomes!

- **Colorful Vegetarian Delights**

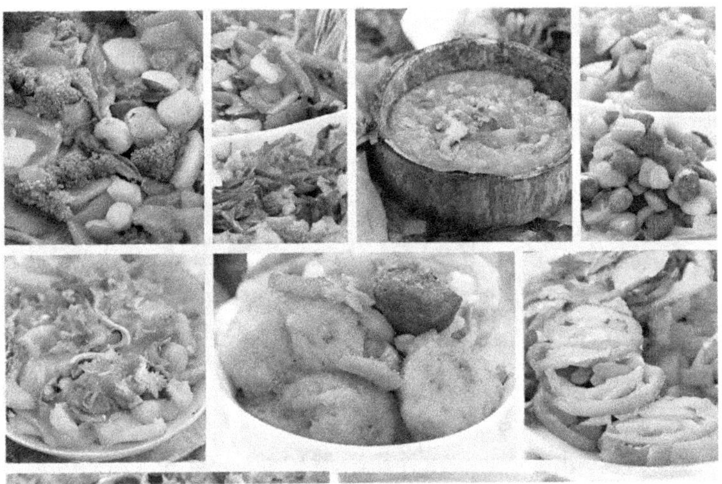

20. Bell peppers stuffed with quinoa and roasted vegetables:

ingredients

- Quartered and seeded four bell peppers
- 1/2 cup black beans, cooked 1/2 cup corn kernels, chopped 1/2 red onion, diced 1/2 zucchini, cooked 1 cup quinoa and
- half a cup cherry tomatoes
- two minced cloves of garlic
- one tsp. cumin
- One teaspoon of chili powder
- To taste, add salt and black pepper.

- To roast, use
olive oil.

Instructions:

1. First, preheat the oven to 400°F, or 200°C.
2. Toss with olive oil, cumin, chili powder, salt, black pepper, and cherry tomatoes. Add zucchini, red onion, and garlic.
3. After 20 to 25 minutes, or until they are soft, roast the veggies.
4. Add the cooked quinoa, black beans, corn, and roasted veggies to a dish and stir.
5. The quinoa and veggie combination should be stuffed within the bell pepper halves.
6. Until the peppers are tender, bake for another 15 to 20 minutes.

21.

Tofu-Sided Rainbow Veggie Stir-Fry:

Ingredients:

- One diced and pressed block of extra-firm tofu
- florets split from one broccoli head
- Slightly chop

- one red bell pepper.
- Thinly slice one yellow bell pepper
- One carrot cut into ribbons
- one cup of trimmed snap peas
- Take three teaspoons of soy sauce.
- Two teaspoons of black sesame oil
- a single spoonful of vinegar made from rice
- A single spoonful of maple syrup
- two minced cloves of garlic
- One ton of ginger, finely chopped green onions, and sesame seeds as garnish

Instructions;

1. Stir-fry the cubes of tofu until golden brown in a wok or big pan. Remove from the way.
2. Add bell peppers, carrots, snap peas, and broccoli to the same pan and stir-fry until crisp-tender.
3. Combine the rice vinegar, ginger, garlic, sesame oil, soy sauce, and maple syrup in a small bowl.
4. Coat the veggies evenly by tossing them with the tofu and sauce.
5. With sesame seeds and green onions as garnish, serve the rainbow stir-fry over cooked rice.

22.   Kale with a Balsamic Dressing:

Ingredients:

- Slicing one pound of fresh mozzarella and four big tomatoes
- new leaves of basil
- Glazed in balsam
- superior-quality olive oil
- To taste, add salt and black pepper.

Instructions:

1. On a serving dish, arrange the tomato and mozzarella slices.
2. Sandwich the mozzarella and tomato slices with a few fresh basil leaves.
3. Pour over olive oil and balsamic glaze.
4. Add black pepper and salt to taste.
5. As a vibrant and reviving salad, serve.

23.   Chilli with Carne and Black Beans:

Ingredients:

- Diced and peeled two big sweet potatoes
- Rinse and drain one can of black beans
- Finely slice one red onion.
- Two tsp. cumin
- One teaspoon of chili powder
- One-teaspoon paprika with smoke
- To taste, add salt and black pepper.
- 8 tortillas made entirely with wheat
- Enchilada sauce in two cups.
- One cup of shredded Mexican mix or cheddar cheese
- fresh cilantro for the garnish

instructions:

1. Preheat the oven to 190°C, or 375°F.
2. Tenderize sweet potatoes by roasting or steaming them.
3. Mash sweet potatoes in a bowl and stir in red onion, cumin, smoked paprika, chili powder, black beans, and salt.
4. Roll each tortilla after spooning the sweet potato and black bean mixture over it, then put it in a roasting tray.
5. Drizzle shredded cheese and enchilada sauce over the rolled tortillas.

6. When the cheese is bubbling and melted, bake it for 20 to 25 minutes.
7. Add some fresh cilantro as a garnish before presenting.

Plant-based foods are beautiful and diverse, as these vibrant vegetarian pleasures highlight. These dishes offer a sensory feast, mixing vivid colors with a variety of filling flavors, whether you're a committed vegetarian or just experimenting with meatless choices. Enjoy making these delectable vegetarian recipes and the process of doing so!

- **Balanced Quinoa and Brown Rice Bowls**

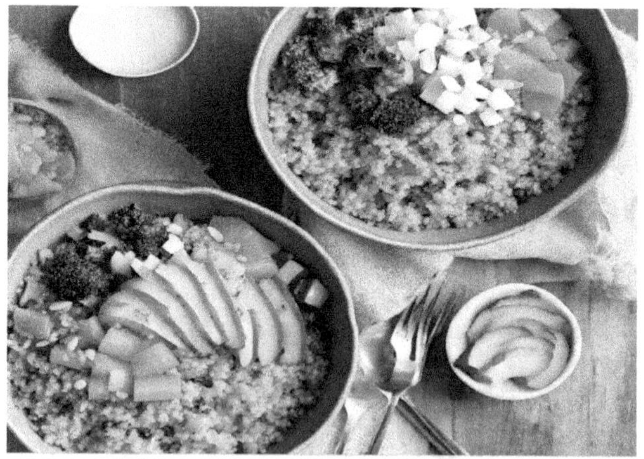

24. Mediterranean Quinoa Bowl:

Ingredients

- One cup of cooked quinoa
- 1/4 cup chopped fresh parsley, diced
- 1/2 red onion, finely chopped
- 1/2 cup Kalamata olives, sliced
- 1/2 cup feta cheese, chopped lemon vinaigrette dressing (olive oil, lemon juice, garlic, salt, and pepper), and
- 1 cup cherry tomatoes

Instructions:

1. Cooked quinoa, cherry tomatoes, cucumber, red onion, olives, feta cheese, and fresh parsley should all be combined in a dish.
2. Add a little drizzle of lemon vinaigrette dressing and gently toss to mix.
3. Savor the flavors of the Mediterranean shortly after serving.

25. Brown rice bowl with teriyaki tofu and vegetables:

Ingredients

- One cup of brown rice, cooked
- One cup of diced firm tofu
- one cup florets of broccoli
- One finely sliced bell pepper and one chopped carrot
- Two tsp soy sauce
- One spoonful of sauce teriyaki
- One tablespoon of sesame oil
- As a garnish, add sesame seeds and green onions.

Instructions:

1. Tofu cubes should be cooked in a wok or pan until golden brown.
2. Stir-fry the broccoli, carrot, and bell pepper in the pan until the veggies are crisp-tender.
3. Combine the sesame oil, teriyaki sauce, and soy sauce in a small bowl.
4. After pouring the sauce over the tofu and veggies, stir to ensure uniform coating.

5. Overcooked brown rice, serve the veggies and teriyaki tofu.

6. garnish with green onions and sesame seeds.

26. Quinoa Bowl with Corn and Spicy Black Beans:

Instructions:

- One cup of cooked quinoa
- One can of washed and drained black beans
- One cup of fresh or frozen corn kernels
- One sliced red bell pepper
- 1 sliced avocado,
- 1/4 cup chopped cilantro, and a lime vinaigrette dressing made with lime juice, olive oil, cumin, chili powder, salt, and pepper

instructions:

1. Cooked quinoa, black beans, corn, avocado, red pepper, and cilantro should all be combined in a dish.

2. Pour in the lime vinaigrette dressing and mix gently.

3. Pour some fresh lime juice over the top of the fiery black bean and corn quinoa dish before serving for an added burst of flavor.

27. Brown rice bowl with grilled chicken and vegetables:

Ingredients

- One cup of brown rice, cooked
- One skinless, boneless grilled chicken breast, sliced
- One cup of cherry tomatoes, cut in half, one zucchini, one yellow squash, and one tablespoon of olive oil
- Seasoning with Italian herbs
- Balsamic glaze to pour over
- For garnish, use fresh basil.

instructions:

1. Sauté cherry tomatoes, yellow squash, and zucchini in olive oil on a grill pan until they are soft.
2. Use some Italian herb seasoning to season the grilled chicken.
3. Arrange the cooked brown rice, sautéed veggies, and grilled chicken in a bowl.

4. Garnish with fresh basil and drizzle with balsamic glaze.
5. Warm brown rice bowl with grilled chicken and vegetables should be served.

These recipes for well-balanced brown rice and quinoa bowls provide a lovely blend of textures and flavors, making them ideal for filling and nutritious meals. Try experimenting with different ingredients and dressings to make bowls that are uniquely personalized for your palate. Savour the benefits of whole foods!

Chapter 4

Snacks and Desserts

- **Smart Snacking for Gallbladder Health**

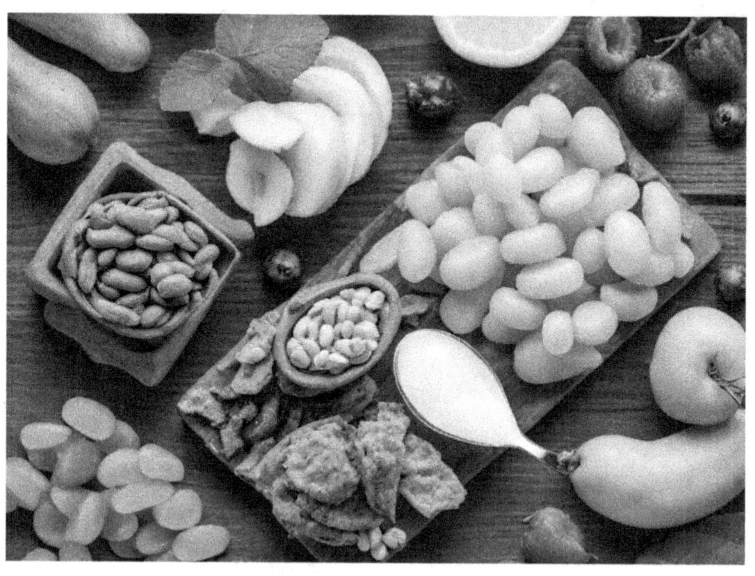

28. Greek Yogurt Parfait:

Ingredients:

- 1 cup Greek yogurt

- Fresh berries (blueberries, strawberries, raspberries)
- 1 tbsp. chia seeds
- 1 tablespoon honey

Instructions:

1. In a glass or dish, top Greek yogurt with fresh berries.
2. Sprinkle chia seeds on each layer.
3. Drizzle honey over the top for sweetness.
4. Enjoy a parfait filled with protein and antioxidants.

29. Avocado with Whole Grain Crackers:

Ingredients:

- 1 ripe avocado
- Whole-grain crackers
- Lemon juice
- Red pepper flakes (optional)

Instructions:

1. Mash the avocado and put it over whole-grain crackers.
2. Squeeze a little lemon juice for added zest.
3. Optionally, add red pepper flakes for a hint of spice.

4. Savor a snack packed with healthy fats and fiber.

30. Roasted Chickpeas:

Ingredients:

- 1 can chickpeas, drained and rinsed
- 1 tablespoon olive oil
- 1 teaspoon cumin
- 1 teaspoon paprika
- Salt and pepper to taste

Instructions:

1. Toss chickpeas with olive oil, cumin, paprika, salt, and pepper.
2. Roast in the oven at 400°F (200°C) for 20–25 minutes until crispy.
3. Allow to cool before munching on these protein-packed goodies.

31. Sliced Apple with Almond Butter:

Ingredients:

- 1 apple, sliced;

- 2 tablespoons almond butter

Instructions:

1. Slice the apple into thin wedges.
2. Dip each slice into almond butter for a delightful blend of sweetness and healthy fats.
3. Enjoy a snack that blends fiber and protein.

33. Vegetable Sticks with Hummus:

Ingredients:

- Carrot sticks, cucumber slices, bell pepper strips
- Hummus for dipping

Instructions:

1. Slice carrots, cucumber, and bell pepper into sticks or slices.
2. Dip each vegetable into hummus for a pleasant and fiber-rich snack.
3. Relish the crunch and vitamin increase.

34. Nut and Seed Mix:

Ingredients:

- Almonds, walnuts, pumpkin seeds, sunflower seeds
- Dried cranberries or raisins (optional)

Instructions:

1. Create a combination of nuts and seeds.
2. Optionally, add dried cranberries or raisins for a hint of sweetness.
3. Portion out for a handy and nutrient-dense snack.

35. Whole Grain Rice Cake with Cottage Cheese:

Ingredients:

- Whole-grain rice cake
- Cottage cheese
- Fresh pineapple chunks (optional)

Instructions:

1. Spread cottage cheese on a whole-grain rice cake.
2. Top with fresh pineapple pieces for additional taste.
3. Delight in a light and pleasant snack.

36. Steamed Edamame:

Ingredients:

- Edamame pods
- Sea salt

Instructions:

1. Steam edamame pods until tender.
2. Sprinkle with sea salt for a simple but healthful snack.
3. Enjoy a plant-based protein boost.

These smart snacking alternatives not only cater to gallbladder health but also provide a range of textures and tastes to keep your taste buds delighted. Incorporate these healthful nibbles into your routine for a balanced and supportive approach to snacking.

- **Guilt-Free Sweet Treats**

Satisfy your needs for sweetness without guilt by indulging in these tasty and health-conscious sweet snacks. Packed with healthful ingredients, these sweets not only pleasure your taste buds but also contribute to your overall well-being.

37. Chocolate Avocado Mousse:

Ingredients:

- 2 ripe avocados
- 1/4 cup cocoa powder
- 1/4 cup maple syrup or honey
- 1 teaspoon vanilla extract
- A pinch of salt

Instructions:

1. Blend avocados, cocoa powder, maple syrup (or honey), vanilla essence, and salt until creamy.
2. Refrigerate for at least 30 minutes before serving.
3. Enjoy a creamy and chocolatey mousse that's packed with healthy fats.

38. Frozen Banana Bites:

Ingredients:

- Bananas, sliced
- Peanut butter or almond butter
- Dark chocolate melted
- Optional toppings: Chopped nuts, shredded coconut

Instructions:

1. Spread peanut butter or almond butter between banana slices.
2. Dip each banana bite in melted dark chocolate.
3. Sprinkle with chopped nuts or shredded coconut.
4. Freeze until the chocolate hardens, then enjoy a frozen, guilt-free pleasure.

39. Greek Yogurt Berry Popsicles:

Ingredients:

1. 1 cup Greek yogurt
2. Mixed berries (strawberries, blueberries, raspberries)
3. 2 tablespoons honey or agave syrup
4. Instructions:
5. Mix Greek yogurt with honey or agave syrup.
6. Layer Greek yogurt and mixed fruit in popsicle molds.
7. Freeze until solid, then relish a delicious and protein-packed popsicle.

40. Chia Seed Pudding Parfait:

Ingredients:

- 1/4 cup chia seeds
- 1 cup almond milk or coconut milk
- 1 teaspoon vanilla extract
- Fresh fruit (berries, mango, kiwi)
- Granola

Instructions:

1. Mix chia seeds, almond milk (or coconut milk), and vanilla essence in a container.
2. Refrigerate overnight to let it thicken.
3. Layer chia pudding with fresh fruit and granola for a parfait that's both delicious and healthful.

41. Baked Cinnamon Apple Chips:

- *Ingredients:*
- Apples, thinly sliced
- Cinnamon
- Optional: A sprinkling of sugar or stevia

Instructions:

1. Preheat the oven to 200°F (93°C).
2. Arrange apple slices on a baking sheet and sprinkle with cinnamon (and optional sugar or stevia).
3. Bake for 2-3 hours until the chips are crunchy.
4. Enjoy a crunchy, naturally sweet snack.

42. Date and Nut Energy Balls:

Ingredients:

- Medjool dates, pitted
- Mixed nuts (almonds, walnuts, and cashews) Unsweetened shredded coconut
- Cocoa powder

Instructions:

1. Blend dates and mixed nuts in a food processor until a sticky dough forms.
2. Roll the mixture into tiny balls.
3. Coat each ball in shredded coconut or cocoa powder.
4. Refrigerate and enjoy these energy-packed sweet treats.

43. Coconut Mango Chia Popsicles:

Ingredients:

- 1 cup coconut milk
- 1 ripe mango, diced
- 2 teaspoons chia seeds
- 1 tablespoon honey or agave syrup

Instructions:

1. Blend coconut milk, sliced mango, chia seeds, and honey (or agave syrup) until smooth.
2. Pour the mixture into popsicle molds and freeze until hardened.
3. Relish a tropical and nutrient-rich frozen delight.

- **Refreshing Fruit-Based Desserts**

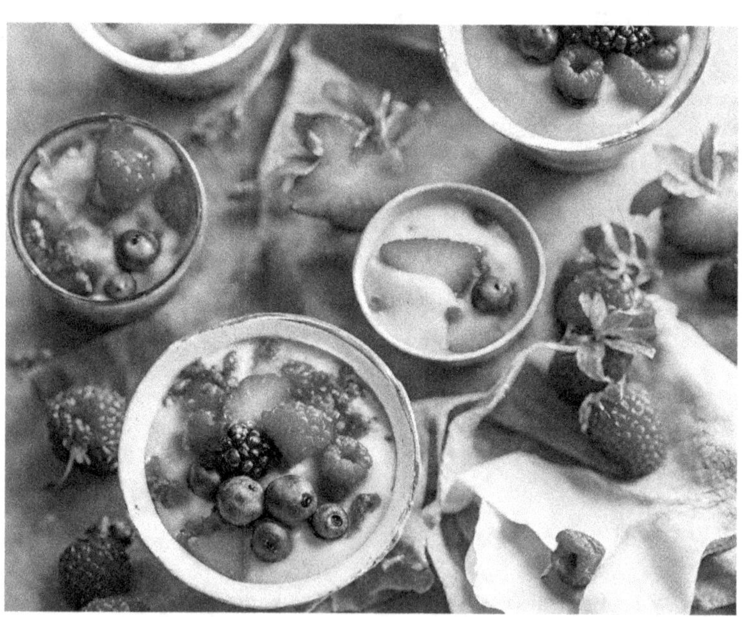

44. Pizza with watermelon:

Ingredients:

- Slicing of thick watermelon
- Coconut yogurt or Greek yogurt?
- Various fresh fruits (mango, kiwi, and berries)
- Mint leaves as a garnish

Guidelines:

1. Top slices of watermelon with yogurt to simulate a pizza "crust."
2. Top with an assortment of fresh fruits.
3. Add some mint leaves as a garnish for a vibrant and revitalizing watermelon pizza.

45. Chia Pudding with Mango Coconut:

Ingredients:

- One cup of chunky mango
- One cup of coconut milk
- One-fourth cup of chia seeds
- Coconut flakes as a garnish

Instructions:

1. Mango chunks and coconut milk should be blended until smooth.

2. Add the chia seeds and chill for a minimum of four hours or overnight.
3. To make a tropical chia pudding, sprinkle coconut flakes on top before serving.

46. Berry Blend Parfait:

- Mixed berries (strawberries, blueberries, raspberries) are the ingredients.
- Vanilla yogurt or Greek yogurt
- Granola Honey to pour over

Instructions:

1. Arrange granola, mixed berries, and Greek yogurt in a glass.
2. Coatings should be repeated until the glass is full.
3. Pour some honey over the berries to create a visually pleasing and tasty parfait.

47. Coconut Pineapple Sorbet:

Ingredients:

- Two cups of frozen pineapple chunks
- half a cup of coconut milk
- One tablespoon of lime juice
- coconut shreds as a garnish

Instructions:

1. Puree the frozen pineapple, lime juice, and coconut milk until smooth.
2. After moving the mixture to a shallow dish, freeze it for three hours or longer.
3. After transferring the sorbet into dishes, sprinkle shredded coconut on top.

48. Yogurt Bites with Berries and Lemons:

Ingredients:

1. Yoghurt made from Greek yoghurt
2. Berries in combination (raspberries, blueberries)
3. Zest of lemons
4. Agave syrup or honey (optional)

Instructions:

1. Combine Greek yogurt with agave syrup or honey, if preferred, and lemon zest.
2. Transfer the yogurt mixture into silicone molds and garnish each with a couple of berries.
3. Pop the frozen yogurt bits out of the freezer when they're firm for a cool snack.

49. Strawberry and Kiwi Salsa:

Ingredients:

- Diced and peeled Kiwi
- Diced strawberries
- Lime juice, chopped fresh mint
- Agave syrup or honey

Instructions:

1. In a dish, mix chopped mint, sliced strawberries, and diced kiwi.
2. Drizzle with agave syrup or honey and lime juice.
3. For a fruity and light dessert, spread over vanilla yogurt or serve as a salsa.

51. Popsicles with Bananas:

Ingredients:

- Halfed and peeled bananas
- Melted dark chocolate
- chopped almonds or flakes of coconut

instructions:

Place popsicle sticks within the halves of bananas.

After dipping each banana into melted dark chocolate, top with coconut flakes or chopped almonds.

Savor a naturally sweet frozen delight once the chocolate has set in the freezer.

Chapter 5

Meal plan

Day 1:

Breakfast:

- Veggie-Packed Egg White Wrap

- Herbal tea or water

Lunch:

- Balanced Quinoa and Brown Rice Bowl with Grilled Chicken and Vegetables

- Mixed green salad with olive oil and lemon dressing

Snack:

- Greek Yogurt Parfait with Fresh Berries and Chia Seeds

Dinner:

- Baked Lemon Herb Tilapia with Steamed Asparagus

- Quinoa Salad with Cherry Tomatoes and Avocado

Day 2:

Breakfast:

- Mango Tango Breakfast Wrap

- Green tea or water

Lunch:

- Sweet Potato and Black Bean Enchiladas

- Cilantro Lime Quinoa

Snack:

- Sliced Apple with Almond Butter

Dinner:

- Grilled Chicken and Vegetable Brown Rice Bowl

- Mixed Berry Parfait for dessert

Day 3:

Breakfast:

- Nutrient-packed oatmeal with Mixed Berries

- Herbal tea or water

Lunch:

- Flavorful Grilled Chicken and Fish Recipes (Choose one)

- Quinoa and Roasted Vegetable Stuffed Bell Peppers

Snack:

- Roasted Chickpeas

Dinner:

- Spicy Black Bean and Corn Quinoa Bowl

- Watermelon Pizza for dessert

Day 4:

Breakfast:

- Light and Satisfying Breakfast Wraps: Avocado and Turkey Wrap

- Green tea or water

Lunch:

- Colorful Vegetarian Delights: Caprese Salad with Balsamic Glaze

- Whole Grain Rice Cake with Cottage Cheese

Snack:

- Mixed Berry Smoothie Bowl

Dinner:

- Cajun Spiced Grilled Chicken Thighs

- Greek Salad with Feta Cheese

Day 5:

Breakfast:

- Energizing Smoothie Bowl with Mixed Fruits and Greek Yogurt

- Herbal tea or water

Lunch:

- Smart Snacking for Gallbladder Health: Vegetable Sticks with Hummus

- Quinoa and Roasted Vegetable Stuffed Bell Peppers

Snack:

- Frozen Banana Bites

Dinner:

- Lemon Herb Grilled Tilapia

- Mango Coconut Chia Pudding for dessert

Day 6:

Breakfast:

- Guilt-Free Sweet Treats: Chocolate Avocado Mousse

- Green tea or water

Lunch:

- Balanced Quinoa and Brown Rice Bowl with Teriyaki Tofu and Vegetables

- Steamed Edamame

Snack:

- Date and Nut Energy Balls

Dinner:

- Flavorful Grilled Chicken and Fish Recipes: Honey Garlic Glazed Salmon

- Mixed Berry Parfait for dessert

Day 7:

Breakfast:

- Smart Snacking for Gallbladder Health: Greek Yogurt Parfait with Fresh Berries and Chia Seeds

- Herbal tea or water

Lunch:

- Colorful Vegetarian Delights: Sweet Potato and Black Bean Enchiladas

- Mediterranean Quinoa Bowl

Snack:

- Pineapple Coconut Sorbet

Dinner:

- Refreshing Fruit-Based Desserts: Kiwi and Strawberry Salsa

- Grilled Lemon Herb Chicken

Remember to listen to your body's signals of hunger and fullness. If any specific food triggers discomfort or digestive issues, consider modifying the meal plan accordingly. This plan emphasizes whole, nutrient-rich foods while minimizing processed and high-fat options to support gallbladder health. Adjustments can be made based on personal preferences and dietary needs. and remember to drink plenty of water throughout the day

Conclusion

Beginning a path to feed and promote the health of your gallbladder is a move that is both praiseworthy and powerful in the direction of overall well-being. This selection of dishes that are safe for the gallbladder makes available a wide variety of alternatives that are both tasty and healthy, demonstrating how flavor and health may be harmoniously combined here.

As you have progressed through the many chapters of this culinary journey, you have come across dishes that highlight lean proteins, healthy fats, and foods that are rich in fiber. These recipes are not only about imposing constraints; rather, they encourage you to immerse yourself in the plethora of flavors that can be found in foods that have been carefully chosen and are healthful.

The purpose of these recipes is to give food that goes beyond just providing sustenance since the authors are aware of the need to maintain a diet that is both balanced and varied. Creating a symphony of flavors that will satisfy your palate and revitalize your body is the goal of the gallbladder-friendly meal plan, which encourages you to enjoy a colorful palette of fruits, vegetables, lean meats, and healthy grains.

Remember that the nutritional requirements of each individual are different, and it is essential to pay attention to the signals that your body sends you. If you are experiencing any pain or have particular dietary issues, talking with a healthcare expert or a certified dietitian may provide you with individualized advise that is customized to your unique situation and requirements.

It is important to note that the route toward supporting gallbladder health is not about deprivation but rather about choosing choices that are educated and thoughtful. Through the incorporation of these dishes into your culinary repertoire, you are adopting a way of life that places equal importance on the pleasure of eating and the health of the body. Continue to explore, adapt, and relish the process of fueling your body with meaningful and pleasurable meals.

May your route to gallbladder health be a joyful and delightful experience, rich with brilliant tastes, healthy foods, and the satisfaction of establishing a balanced and thoughtful attitude to eating. Cheers to your health and the fascinating gastronomic experiences that lie ahead!

Sustaining a Gallbladder-Friendly Lifestyle

Embarking on a gallbladder-friendly lifestyle takes more than simply following a series of recipes; it's a commitment to long-term well-being and a thoughtful approach to how you fuel your body. As you continue on your path, consider the following tips to preserve a gallbladder-friendly lifestyle:

1. Mindful Eating:

- ❖ Pay heed to your body's cues of hunger and fullness.
- ❖ Eat gently, appreciating each mouthful, and be present throughout meals to aid digestion.

2. Stay Hydrated:

- ❖ Adequate hydration improves digestion and helps prevent the production of gallstones.
- ❖ Strive to drink lots of water throughout the day.

3. Embrace Variety:

- ❖ Incorporate a varied mix of fruits, vegetables, lean meats, and healthy grains into your meals.
- ❖ Experiment with diverse tastes and textures to make your meals intriguing.

4. Monitor Portion Sizes:

- ❖ Be cautious of portion amounts to prevent overeating, which may put pressure on your gallbladder.
- ❖ Listen to your body's instincts and eat until you're satisfied, not too full.

5. Choose healthy fats:

- ❖ Opt for sources of healthy fats such as avocados, nuts, seeds, and olive oil.
- ❖ Limit saturated and trans fats present in processed and fried meals.

6. Maintain a healthy weight:

- ❖ Achieving and maintaining a healthy weight is vital for gallbladder health.
- ❖ Incorporate regular physical exercise into your routine to improve your overall well-being.

7. Minimize processed foods:

- ❖ Reduce consumption of processed and refined foods, which may lead to gallbladder troubles.
- ❖ Choose entire, nutrient-dense foods wherever feasible.

8. Monitor trigger foods:

- ❖ Pay attention to how your body responds to particular meals.
- ❖ Identify and avoid trigger foods that may cause pain or digestive difficulties.

9. Regular physical activity:

- ❖ Engage in regular exercise to boost overall health and assist in maintaining a healthy weight.
- ❖ Consult with a healthcare expert to discover the best-suited fitness plan for you.

10. Regular check-ups:

* Schedule frequent check-ups with your healthcare professional to monitor your gallbladder health.
* Discuss any concerns or changes in your symptoms with your healthcare staff.

11. Personalized Approach:

* Everyone's body is unique; what works for one person may not work for another.
* Tailor your food choices to your unique requirements, and speak with healthcare specialists for specialized recommendations.

12. Be patient and positive.

* Adopting a gallbladder-friendly lifestyle is a gradual process.
* Be patient with yourself, enjoy tiny wins, and have a good attitude about your health journey.